Cannabis
And
Healing

VENERINA CONTI

DEDICATION

Dedicated to the most beautiful and strong person I have ever had the honour of knowing from birth till death, Linsey Dagger (1976 - 2010,) my friend and adopted sister. Her struggle with cancer and her will to survive, long after her doctor's predictions, inspires me to live daily and to help others whenever, wherever and however I can. Her light still shines bright in my heart like a beacon that guides me towards a better me for the sake of others.

If only one person takes note of what I've written and reaps any benefit at all, I will honestly be able to say that, for me, Linsey's death was not in vain. Gone but never forgotten. Loved forever.

CONTENTS

DISCLAIMER

Dear beautiful human being,

Welcome to my booklet.

Thank you for purchasing it and taking the time to read it. I would like to strongly stress that everything written herein, although thoroughly researched and almost entirely based on scientific fact, sourced from reputable sites and publications, it is still based on my own personal opinion.

I am not an authority on the cannabis plant nor its healing potential. Nor do I claim to be.

My only intention is to make you more aware of the beneficial properties of medicinal cannabis and maybe dispel a few myths. You do not have to agree with anything I say. In fact, I would encourage you to do your own research and come to your own conclusions.

My sole motivation for writing this booklet is because I lost a dear friend, more like an adopted sister, to cancer back in 2010 just before her 34th birthday, which would have been on the launch date of this booklet. They say that hindsight is a wonderful thing but I just wish I'd known then what I know now.

I am not claiming that cannabis will cure you in any way, shape or form. However, I would ask that you keep an open mind when approaching the subject.

No disease will ever be cured using cannabis alone. It's necessary to follow a good alkaline nutritional program and have a healthy lifestyle where work and relaxation are equally balanced. Stress should be reduced to a minimum and it's always good to meditate or take up yoga.

Science has proven that cannabis can help in many ways if it's taken correctly. There are also many testimonials, on the Internet, about how cannabis has helped people to varying degrees. So, please take a little time to check them out. You can find them on youtube or through any search engine by typing in: Cannabis healing testimonials.

A word of caution. All cannabis is not the same and the cannabis you find on the street is genetically modified. So, if purchasing cannabis at all, please ensure that you get medical grade or grow it yourself, organically, to avoid an over saturation of THC or pesticides and other farming chemicals.

Be safe, be happy and be healthy!

One Global Love

1 INTRODUCTION

When you think about Cannabis and its uses, what do you think about? Illegal drugs? Junkies? Old hippies? People sat around in communes getting high? Crime and drug cartels? - well, think again.

It can, technically, be all of those things. Yet, Cannabis is so much more than just the recreational drug or the bad publicity it's often given by the media to serve corporate agendas. At this point, it's important to remember that, nowadays, the media is no longer unbiased. It's very much sponsored by the highest bidder and the pharmaceutical companies have a massive financial interest in you buying their "legal" drugs.

You should, also, be aware that many university studies, and nearly all research that is published in the mainstream media, are bogus. These "so called" studies are backed by sponsors who have an interest in steering public opinion the way these big corporations want them to go and pharmaceuticals do not want you to stop buying their products.

Pharmaceutical companies will resort to any measure needed to keep the Cannabis healing properties still relatively unknown in the mainstream. They will resort to telling you it's bad. They will convince you it's addictive, which it's not. In fact, most legal drugs that you buy over the pharmacy counter will create much more of a dependency than Cannabis. Codeine, which is an active ingredient in pain killers such as Migraleve, is a highly addictive substance that, over a period of time, used in even moderate doses, can cause dependency. Hence, in Portugal, Italy and Spain, you need a prescription to purchase Migraleve and other pharmaceuticals that contain codeine. However, in the UK Migraleve and other medication, containing codeine, can be freely bought over the counter at a local chemist.

Cigarettes create more of a dependency than cannabis and can be legally purchased at many establishments. They're advertised wittingly and unwittingly as sexy, trendy and cool. Yet, they remain one of the main causes of cancer and deaths through cancer.

Through carefully drafted press releases, corporations like the big pharmaceuticals, will use mainstream media to instill fear in you with their false information about cannabis and its effects on the human body or brain. They will resort to paying backhanders to governments to pass laws to prohibit you from being able to get legal access to the plant. Although, it is worth noting that, since 2015, the use of medicinal and recreational cannabis has slowly become legal in many US states and several countries like Spain, Jamaica, India, Portugal and Mexico among others. Hopefully, many more will follow suit.

A word of caution though. Before you rush out and buy cannabis plants to grow, please check your country or state's legislation.

Coming back to the topic of the illegality of cannabis, history has taught us that enforcing prohibition laws serves two great purposes. The first is psychological. If we believe something is prohibited by law, and we hold faith in the "good" intentions of our governments to look out for us, then we will automatically believe the prohibited substance must be bad.

The general rationale is, if it was good it would not be illegal, right? Since the majority of us have, to varying degrees, the wish to believe that authority and authoritative figures know best, we believe without questioning.

I might add that, since we all lead quite egocentric lives, and I don't mean that in a bad way, we all tend to get caught up in our own worlds and routines that we don't think to question anything until the need arises or it touches us personally. In many ways that can make us quite apathetic towards various issues going on in the world. In my personal experience, I have also found that many people still consider cannabis a taboo subject of conversation.

The second main purpose of prohibition is of economical interest. The more a substance is illegal, the greater its black market value and it would be very naive to think governments do not reap rewards from black markets.

Given this insight, it's safe to say that if we all turned to cannabis as one of many alternative forms of healing, the pharmaceutical companies would lose billions every year and so would our governments. What might be more shocking to know is that cancer patients alone rake in 100 billion dollars a year for pharmaceutical companies.

One of the main obstructions and challenges still faced by the world of alternative medicine, as I see it, is overcoming pre-conditioning the general public has been, and still is being, subjected to. What I mean by this is how people have become so conditioned into thinking conventional medicine is the only way. The truth is, pharmaceutical companies employ the best market researchers, publicists and psychologists who know how to design advertising campaigns that play to our deepest fears and most sensitive emotions. They wittingly and unwittingly make us buy. In essence, we have been manipulated into a "legal drug" culture.

Over the years, practitioners have defined a label for every condition and pharmaceuticals have responded with a pill for every label. We are, falsely, led to believe the only solution are their legal drugs. Yet, nowadays, it's probably fairer to say that conventional medicine is no longer about healing. It's about a multi billion dollar corporate business. In fact, realistically speaking, legal drugs do not actually treat the root cause of illness, they just mask the symptoms.

For example, when someone suffers a headache or migraine, they pop a pill and the pain disappears for a few hours, a day or a week, but if the root cause of the headache is not addressed, which might be stress or an intolerance to a particular food or blood pressure issues, the headache will return and, again, more pills will be popped. The headache or migraine sufferer becomes dependent on drugs for relief but the actual cause is never addressed. So, relief is only a temporary state.

Unfortunately, we live in a time where we want quick fixes and immediate results. The fast relief "Pill popping" culture fits nicely into this paradigm and pharmaceuticals are capitalising on it.

Another example might be diabetes. The drugs given to diabetics are prescribed to help patients "manage" their condition. They artificially adjust blood sugar levels but they don't actually cure anything. They don't address the root of the problem nor do they restore proper functioning of the pancreas. All they do is make life a little easier for a while.

The fact remains though, that, according to a fact sheet published by the World Health Organisation (WHO), over 422 million people died from diabetes in 2014; presumably while taking legally prescribed medication through their doctor. And, according to an investigation carried out by Visiongain, the diabetic market is set to reach an estimated worth of 55,3 billion dollars in 2017. So, as you can probably see by now, it's definitely not in the pharmaceutical companies' interest that people be completely cured.

Similarly, for any type of dis-ease in the body, we resort to popping pills to masquerade the pain so we can function on some level of normality, whatever that may be, and all the while the pharmaceutical companies are cashing in on it.

According to statistics published by the World Health Organisation, the pharmaceutical companies are worth 300 billion dollars. Apparently, that figure is set to rise to 400 billion dollars within the next few years with the onset of more diseases and the rising number of people on a global scale.

I'd like to, also, add that pharmaceutical companies, especially in the United States, are known to be huge political campaign contributors. According to Open Secrets - the centre for responsive politics, in 2012, the pharmaceutical companies donated just over 50 billion dollars to political campaigning. And, although, the pharmaceuticals have a predilection for supporting the Republicans, who received 58% of said funds, the Democrats benefitted as well from 42% of the very same contributions. So, theoretically, it doesn't matter who wins the elections, the pharmaceutical companies are behind both parties and their strength increases with every passing election.

In 2008, when President Obama was elected into the White House, pharmaceutical companies signed contracts worth billions with the US government, which doubled or tripled their net worth, literally, overnight. According to Forbes, with the introduction of the Obamacare plan, the pharmaceuticals were set to earn an estimated 45 billion dollars.

With so much money involved, perhaps now, you can understand why pharmaceutical companies want to protect their income at all costs.

"At all costs" are the key words here. When it comes to protecting their income, the pharmaceutical companies are quite unscrupulous. In 2009, there was a scandal when someone leaked a pharmaceutical hit-list, which was meant to intimidate or annihilate practitioners, holistic or otherwise, who would not adhere to their policies and sell their products. In true dictatorial fashion, the pharmaceuticals have tried to silence anyone who speaks out against them.

Since 2009, many fellow naturopaths, chiropractors and doctors with holistic training have mysteriously died or disappeared and in 2015, 29 natural doctors were poisoned during a holistic conference held in Germany. Some died and some were left in a critical condition.

You might argue that the pharmaceuticals had nothing to do with these events. You may even argue they were isolated attacks. Whether, or not, the pharmaceutical companies were directly, or indirectly, involved in any of these occurrences is debatable, because there is no concrete evidence for or against this argument, but it does seem to be too much of a coincidence.

As a curious sideline, when I went looking for my original sources of information on the Internet, that I read back in 2009, I noted the website referring to the 2009 hit-list scandal, and subsequent court case in Australia, had been removed. However, I did come across an interesting website with a comprehensive list of *Persecuted (and murdered) doctors, health professionals* at www.whale.to

Just last year, in 2015, Novartis were being sued by the US government; accused of 80,000 offences related to bribing doctors into selling their products. I don't see any of those offences being punished.

Coming back to the topic of cannabis, another interesting fact about pharmaceuticals is that, instead of using the wholesome cannabis plant in a controlled environment, for years they have been experimenting with ways to synthesize it.

In Portugal, in 2015, a pharmaceutical company called Bial succeeded; creating a synthetic cannabinoid based painkiller that was/is intended to treat anxiety and motor function disorders associated with neurodegenerative diseases.

In January 2016, in Rennes (France), a laboratory called Biotrial ran an experiment with this synthetic drug; using 8 healthy participants. 2 participants were given placebos and the remaining 6 were given varying dosages of the synthetic drug. The outcome was that, out of the 6 who were given the drug, 1 suffered irreversible brain damage and the other 5 were taken into intensive care in a critical condition.

As far as I'm aware, to date, there have never been any reported deaths linked to the use of Cannabis. Naturally cannabis users have died. We all will one day, but there have been no deaths reported as a direct consequence of using cannabis. There probably never will be either.

The outstandingly good news is that, according to a research paper called *Substituting cannabis for prescription drugs, alcohol and other substances among medical cannabis patients: The impact of contextual factors* carried out by the Centre for Addictions Research of BC - University of Victoria in Canada - out of 410 people surveyed, 80.3% said they would willingly substitute prescription medication with cannabis. So, more and more people seem to be opening up to the healing properties of this ancient plant.

So, is cannabis safe to use? Yes. Do you have to smoke it? No. In fact, as you read through this booklet, you'll probably be surprised to discover that there are several different ways to use cannabis and each serves its own purpose.

The longer I live, the more I discover that healing exists all around us in nature. We just need to know what it is we are looking for, where to look for it and how to harness the beneficial properties each plant holds.

Cannabis, despite its reputation as a recreational drug, is just another gift from mother nature in the form of a plant with many beneficial healing properties.

2 A BRIEF HISTORY OF CANNABIS

Have you ever wondered where the Cannabis plant came from? Well, according to the book: "Marihuana: The First Twelve Thousand Years," it appears to have originated from areas we know, nowadays, as Mongolia and southern Siberia about 12,000 years ago, which makes it one of the oldest plants known to human beings.

I should mention here that, nowadays, there are different varieties of cannabis. There is cannabis sativa, cannabis indica and cannabis ruderalis. Each variety has been developed to have different characteristics and a different level of cannabinoid content. The variety that contains the least cannabinoid content, and the one everyone is probably more familiar with, is called hemp.

According to Abel, dating back as far as 10,000 years ago, the Chinese used hemp in their pottery work and as a sturdy fibre for making home woven fabrics.

"The discovery that twisted strands of fiber were much stronger than individual strands was followed by developments in the arts of spinning and weaving fibers into fabric—innovations that ended man's reliance on animal skins for clothing. Here, too, it was hemp fiber that the Chinese chose for their first homespun garments. So important a place did hemp fiber occupy in ancient Chinese culture that the Book of Rites (second century B.c.) ordained that out of respect for the dead, mourners should wear clothes made from hemp fabric, a custom followed down to modern times. While traces of early Chinese fabrics have all but disappeared, in 1972 an ancient burial site dating back to the Chou dynasty (1122-249 B.c.) was discovered. In it were fragments of cloth, some bronze containers, weapons, and pieces of jade. Inspection of the cloth showed it to be made of hemp, making this the oldest preserved specimen of hemp in existence."

Abel goes on to mention how the Chinese also used hemp for making shoes and, subsequently, paper. It is presumed that, in the 9th century AD, through the invention of paper and with the Battle of Samarkand between the Chinese and the Arabs, the Arab world came to learn about hemp and began to grow the cannabis plant in their own regions.

Throughout history, in countries like India, Tibet and Persia, cannabis was also used for magical, religious and medicinal purposes. In times gone by, when magic, superstition and illness all went hand in hand, people created amulets and charms with the plant and burned the leaves in cleansing rituals and shamanic practices. Tibetan Lamas would burn the plant to ward off evil spirits. In India, hemp was considered sacred because it was thought to be a plant directly connected to Shiva.It was only later on, with the advent of a systematic practice of medicine, that the Chinese started to use cannabis as a natural anesthetic and a medicinal plant.

Of course, after that, with wars, the rise of colonies and the discovery of new worlds, cannabis slowly found its way around the globe and began to take home in all countries.

In his book, Abel gives a detailed account of how cannabis came to be regarded so highly in each country and how it came to travel throughout the world. It is readily available on the Internet in a pdf format and I've added a link to it in the references section. So, if you would like to learn more, it's definitely worth a read.

The question is: *If cannabis had been used for so long, by so many cultures, how and why did it become illegal?*

According to the Independent Drug Monitoring Unit, in 1928, the United Kingdom brought into force the League of Nations 1925 Dangerous Drugs Act that was devised to combat the problem of foreign immigrants using opium and cocaine on homeland soil, which was causing bad press. Although relatively little was known about the uses of cannabis, and the hemp used in manufacturing was never thought of as cannabis, nobody really lobbied for or against the plant. Apparently, it was just added to the act because Egypt and Turkey requested it to be. They deemed the plant a dangerous drug, nobody bothered to investigate it, nobody really cared either way and so, it became illegal in all 57 nations that formed the League.

In the United States it became illegal owing to bad press and the anti-cannabis campaigning carried out by Harry J Aslinger who, during the 1930s, was head of the Federal Bureau for Narcotics. For more detailed information, please take a while to read the whole article on the Independent Drug Monitoring site. I have added their link in the reference section at the back of this ebook.

In modern times, you will find there are many countries like Spain, and several US states, that have now legalised growing and using cannabis for personal consumption. Although, selling it is still strictly prohibited and even though personal cannabis consumption is legal, you will find there are restrictions, in place, on the amount of plants you are allowed to grow. You might find you also need a special permit to grow as is required in Spain, for example. So, please do check your local country's laws before you decide to set up a cannabis farm.

For further information, I found a very humour filled article on Thrillist that puts things into perspective. You can find the link at the back of this book.

3 CANNABIS THE PLANT

As I mentioned in an earlier chapter, Cannabis and its uses date back at least 12000 years. You may be surprised to know that between 1850 and 1942 cannabis was actually listed in the United States Pharmacopeia as a remedy for nausea, rheumatoid and labour pain. Of course, then it became an illegal substance and banned.

Through the sheer perseverance of its defenders, over the last three or four decades, a lot of scientific research has been conducted, globally, in carefully monitored environments. Slowly but surely, scientists from all over the world are discovering the medical benefits of the cannabis plant. Hence many countries now legalising the use of medical marihuana.

More importantly, these scientific discoveries are being made public knowledge via research publications in scientific journals, abstracts appearing on the world wide web and scientists making their own documentaries.

With the huge growth of the Internet over the last couple of decades and the growing use of smart phones with direct access to the Internet, information is being shared at an astounding rate in, almost, all four corners of the world. Every day, people just like you and me can post whatever they want, whenever they want from wherever they are. So, if you do a little research, you will find an infinity of web pages, blogs and youtube videos that stand testimony to the beneficial healing properties of cannabis in all its forms and uses.

But, why is Cannabis so beneficial and what are its properties? Let's start with the properties.

First of all, you should know that the cannabis plant can be either male or female. More to the point, the Cannabis plant produces either male flowers known as *staminates* or female flowers known as *pistillates*. Some Cannabis plants do produce both male and female flowers at different locations on the plant. However it's, apparently, very rare to find a plant that has male and female flowers growing together in unison at the same location on the plant.

Without getting too botanically and chemically technical, for the purposes of this book it suffices to know that the outer part of the female flower is where terpenoids and cannabinoids are produced among other chemical compounds; 800 in total.

Terpenoids are also known as, or sometimes referred to as *isoprenoids* and are responsible for giving plants their particular smell, flavour or colour. Terpenoids or Isoprenoids are not exclusive to the cannabis plant. In fact, they are a fundamental ingredient for the production of essential oils used in Aromatherapy. They are what is extracted into the oil to give it its strong smell like, for example, eucalyptus, lavender or lemon.

Cannabinoids, on the other hand, are exclusive to the cannabis plant or so it was originally thought. I will explain that later.

Apparently there are about 85 different types of cannabinoids in a single flower. However, it's important to note that only some are psychoactive; not all.
The two main types of cannabinoids people talk about are: tetrahydrocannabinol (THC,) which contains psychoactive properties and cannabidiol (CBD,) which is not psychoactive. In fact, CBD has the opposite effect. It serves to calm a person down from the effects of the THC.

Above, I mentioned that it was originally thought that cannabinoids were exclusive to the cannabis plant, yet research carried out during the 1980s brought to life what is now known as our endocannabinoid system. Basically, scientists discovered that the human body produces its own set of cannabinoids that are responsible for our emotions, our movements, our appetite and our sleep patterns. The prefix endo just means produced internally.

These natural cannabinoids, found in our bodies, interact with two specific receptors known as CB1 that are found in our nervous system, on our nerve endings and in our brain, and CB2 that are located in our immune system.

Explained as simply as possible, a receptor is a protein molecule that can be both inside and outside a cell membrane. Its function is to receive chemical signals from outside the cell, transmit them to the cell and cause that cell to respond in some way.

So what happens when we ingest cannabis? Well, the cannabinoids from the cannabis plant enter our body and link together with our natural cannabinoids. This causes a reaction that then affects our mood, sleep, appetite, movements, emotions, thinking process, memory and our body's ability to fight off disease and naturally heal itself. This is why many people who use cannabis remark that they have more appetite, or they feel more relaxed or they sleep better. In other words, the cannabis works together with our own cannabinoids.

4 CANNABIS – THERAPEUTIC BENEFITS

According to an article published in the British Journal of Clinical Pharmacology, 2012, which I've broken up into sections, cannabis:

" ... *has been reported to have anti-inflammatory properties, thus being useful for neuroinflammatory disorders, including multiple sclerosis for which CBD combined with Δ^9-THC (Sativex®) has been recently licenced as a symptom-relieving agent for the treatment of spasticity and pain.*

Based on its anticonvulsant properties, CBD has been proposed for the treatment of epilepsy, and also for the treatment of sleep disorders based on its capability to induce sleep.

CBD has antitumoural properties that explain its potential against various types of cancer.

CBD has recently shown an interesting profile for psychiatric disorders, for example, it may serve as an antipsychotic and be a promising compound for the treatment of schizophrenia, but it also has potential as an anxiolytic and antidepressant, thus being also effective for other psychiatric disorders.

Lastly, based on the combination of its anti-inflammatory and anti-oxidant properties, CBD has been demonstrated to have an interesting neuroprotective profile as indicated by results obtained through intense preclinical research into numerous neurodegenerative disorders, in particular the three disorders addressed in this review, neonatal ischaemia (CBD alone), Huntington's disease (HD) (CBD combined with Δ⁹-THC as in Sativex®) or Parkinson's disease (PD) (CBD probably combined with the phytocannabinoid Δ⁹-tetrahydrocannabivarin, Δ⁹-THCV), work that has recently progressed to the clinical area in some specific cases.

The neuroprotective potential of CBD for the management of certain other neurodegenerative disorders, e.g. Alzheimer's disease, stroke and multiple sclerosis, has also been investigated in studies that have yielded some positive result"

Taking into consideration the article above, let's take a closer look at why cannabis is considered an effective treatment for the diseases mentioned. I would like to point out that it's not my intention to go into great depth nor to give you a detailed account of each. I just want to give you a synthesis that might encourage you to do your own research and come to your own conclusions.

Multiple sclerosis

Multiple sclerosis is the name given to the auto immune disease caused by an inflammation of the myelin sheaths around neurons in the spine and in the brain. The consequences are muscle spasms and spasticity.

What does this mean in layman's terms? Basically, our body's have their own army of cells dedicated to defending us from outside attacks from viruses, for example. This army of protective cells is referred to as our immune system and the cells are, also, known as our immune cells.

In sufferers of multiple sclerosis, instead of protecting the body, these immune cells attack the body's own central nervous system. The nerves (neurons) in our central nervous system are surrounded by a protective cover, which is called a myelin sheath.

When the immune cells attack the nervous system, they cause an inflammation of this protective cover. Over a period of time, this inflammation leads to long term, irreversible, damage; causing MS sufferers to experience short sharp bursts of temporary muscle pain (spasms) and sharp contractions of the muscles, also described as a feeling of tightness (spasticity.) The body's whole muscular and skeletal system is affected, which leads to mobility problems, causes a great deal of pain, an inability to sleep and, in some cases, depression. Of course, the severity of symptoms will differ from sufferer to sufferer.

Clinical trials concluded that, due to the CB1 receptors I mentioned in an earlier chapter, Cannabis slowed down the immune response and thereby reduced the inflammation of the myelin sheath; reducing the severity of spasms, spasticity and the amount of pain sufferers felt. As a consequence of the reduction in pain, MS sufferers slept better and had more control over their motor functions.

Epilepsy

Epilepsy is a neurological disorder that, due to certain electrical activity in the brain, causes the sufferer to have sudden seizures, which causes them to pass out and be unconscious for a certain amount of time. It's worth noting here that not all seizures are the same and that one person may suffer a series of different seizures.

On the Internet, you can find a wealth of testimonials from parents who have given their children varying doses of liquid cannabis extract high in CBD (cannabidiol) and low in THC (the psychoactive ingredient.) The results obtained, for controlling seizures, are amazing and I would encourage anyone to watch a few video documentaries on youtube as well.

Knowing what we know now about cannabis and its potential to protect nerve cells and brain activity, it is understandable how it can control seizures.

However, as I was conducting my research for this booklet, I was faced with the reality that, even though, as the article above states: *"CBD has been proposed for the treatment of epilepsy,"* to this date, May 2016, there is no real clinical research and the are no real clinical trial results available. All the results I found referred to uncontrolled studies or to parents and epilepsy sufferers who are auto medicating.

Perhaps now that medical cannabis has become legal in many places, new research will come to light in the very near future. One can hope!

Cancer

I was going to write a huge chapter on the benefits of cannabis in the treatment of cancer but then, I discovered an amazing website: Higher

Perspectives.com. If you've never visited the page, you really should. The people who run the site have gone to a lot of trouble to compile an amazingly comprehensive collection of links to scientific research that promotes the healing benefits of cannabis in patients with all different types of cancer.

In the Appendix section of this booklet, I have posted just a few of those links for you to take a look at. You will find them appropriately labelled under their own section. However, they are all worthy of a read.

If you use the search engines, you will also find the Internet is full of testimonials by people who have auto administered cannabis for the treatment of their cancer or they have administered it, in some form, to a loved one. You can see, first hand, the amazing results they have obtained. Youtube is another place you will find hundreds, if not thousands, of testimonials.

The questions remains though: "Why does Cannabis work in treating cancer patients?"

To answer that question, you need to understand how cancer and the cells work. First of all, you should know that all of us have cancer. Since we are living beings made up of cells, any one of the cells can become a mutant at any time. It's just that in most cases, our body's own defence mechanism finds them, doesn't recognise them as being good and kills them off without you being aware of anything happening at all. The human body really is incredible. It's only in cases where the body doesn't recognise the alien nature of the cell or it's unable to kill it that cancer, as the disease we know, comes into being.

Another thing you should know is that every cell membrane has what are known as interconvertible sphingolipids. Interconvertible is self explanatory. Sphingolipids, on the other hand, are fat soluble substances that are components of a living cell. They reside mainly in the cell membrane and they are responsible for receiving transmissions to the cell and recognition of the cell itself. Cancer research, conducted in recent years, suggests there is evidence Sphingolipids are, actually, responsible for the life and death of a cell.

Some Sphingolipids are more simple than others that are more complex. The simple ones are known as ceramides. Of course, the chemistry of all that I'm mentioning goes way beyond my explanation, here, but I want to keep things as simple as possible so that anyone who is not a chemist can understand.

In cancer research it has been found that ceramides can either proliferate the growth of cancer cells or they can destroy a cancerous cell; depending on other important factors. According to the research paper *Diverse functions of ceramide in cancer cell death and proliferation < ... there are diverse functions of endogenously generated ceramides,* *which seem to be context dependent, regulated by subcellular/membrane localization and presence/absence of direct targets of these lipid molecules.>*

So, what we know is, if there is a healthy production of ceramides cancer cells can be destroyed by the body itself. If, on the other hand, there is a defect in the generation of ceramides, along with other factors, cancer can grow freely.

So, how does cannabis fit in to all this?

Well, we saw in an earlier chapter that cannabinoids from the cannabis plant are similar to natural cannabinoids found in our own bodies. We looked at the two different types of cannabinoids in our bodies, CB1 and CB2, and their functions. We also found that once cannabis has been ingested, the cannabinoids from the plant bind with our own cannabinoids. In doing so, they activate either our immune system or our cell messaging system.

Our immune system is designed to protect us, as you know, but sometimes stress, viruses, illness or other causes can weaken our defences. So, what our bodies can't produce to defend us is provided by the external cannabinoids.

According to the article *How Cannabis Oil works to kill Cancer Cells* by Dennis Hill, *It is known that THC and CBD are biomimetic to anandamide, that is, the body can use both interchangeably. Thus, when stress, injury, or illness demand more from endogenous anandamide than can be produced by the body, its mimetic exocannabinoids are activated. If the stress is transitory, then the treatment can be transitory. If the demand is sustained, such as in cancer, then treatment needs to provide sustained pressure of the modulating agent on the homeostatic systems.*

Huntington's Disease

Huntington's is a disease that causes degeneration of the brain and is usually inherited. It's caused by gene mutations that are often inherited. As the disease progresses, a sufferer begins to lose full cognitive functioning. It also causes sudden jerky movements and repetitive behaviour. As it stands, conventional medicine offers no cure for Huntington's disease. Doctors may prescribe anti-depressants, anti-inflammatories but with little results.

According to the study *Neuroprotective effects of phytocannabinoid-based medicines in experimental models of Huntington's disease*, clinical trials with rats induced with cannabis proved to be effective in reducing the physical symptoms as well as inducing a state of relaxation. This study was carried out in 2011, so no doubt nowadays, with the legalization of cannabis in many countries, there are probably "human" trials taking place as I type.

Parkinson's Disease

As you may, or may not, know, Parkinson's is a progressive debilitating disease that affects the nervous system and the nerve cells found in the brain; especially those responsible for movement.

It is important to note that some of our nerve cells (neurons) produce a chemical substance known as dopamine that signals to our brain movements within our body. The more dopamine creating cells we have, the more movement is possible. Similarly, the less dopamine producing cells we have, the less movement is possible.

In Parkinson's disease there is a slow, but progressive, degeneration of the nerve cells until they die out. As these nerve cells die, the production of dopamine is also, naturally, reduced, which leads to an impairment of movement and other pathologies that are related to motor functioning in the body. Swallowing becomes difficult. Walking can become almost impossible. Individuals with this disease will suffer extreme pain due to stiffness in the body. Some may suffer depression and an inability to sleep.

To this day little is known about the exact causes of Parkinson's, although there is much speculation. Some say genes and the environment are responsible. Others claim that genetic mutation may play a part. It has also been suggested that pesticides and chemicals may be a direct cause.

However, there is no specifically known cause. Thus, there is also no known cure. Conventional medication may ease the pain and help movement to some degree but it does not cure.

As with many studies I have already referred to, it has been found that cannabinoids provide a form of protection for the nerve cells. So, in the specific case of Parkinson's, cannabis can slow the progression of the disease by decreasing the rate at which nerve cells degenerate. This, then, slows down the reduction of dopamine and allows the body to retain a certain amount of mobility.

As with the studies on Multiple sclerosis, Parkinson's sufferers using cannabis, as an alternative treatment, found they slept better and had a significant reduction in pain.

Alzheimer's

Pretty much like Huntington's, Alzheimers is a disease that causes a degeneration of the neural tissue in the brain. Unlike Huntington's, it's not inherited. It normally affects people over the age of 65. Their mental and physical health deteriorates to such a degree that they become incapable of looking after themselves.

In January 2016 a research paper called *Safety and Efficacy of Medical Cannabis Oil for Behavioral and Psychological Symptoms of Dementia: An-Open Label, Add-On, Pilot Study* published the conclusive results from a trial involving 11 human volunteers; suffering with alzheimers. Only 10 patients concluded the trial but the beneficial results were considerable in all 10. They suffered less anxiety, less moodiness, less aggression and slept better.

Glaucoma

Glaucoma is a disease that affects the eyes. It's caused by damage to the optical nerve and can lead to side blindness or complete loss of vision. One of the main causes of Glaucoma is, what is known as, Intraocular pressure (IOP) or, in layman's terms, a high amount of pressure in the eyes. Another cause is the lack of blood flow to the optical nerve.

Research concluded that as much as cannabis is effective, to some degree, in lowering intraocular pressure, it also lowers the body's blood pressure, which means there is less blood flow to the eyes. This, as I mentioned earlier is actually one of the causes of glaucoma. So, the benefits reaped from using Cannabis are, in fact, counteracted. Another drawback found, during clinical trials, was that the intraocular pressure only lowered for 3 to 4 hours. The conclusions are that more research is needed in this area.

5 FACTS AND MYTHS

Myth No. 1 - The use of Cannabis causes memory loss and brain damage.

Fact -   Cannabis does not cause memory loss nor brain damage.

According to the research paper, ***Impact of cannabidiol on the acute memory and psychotomimetic effects of smoked cannabis: naturalistic study: naturalistic study [corrected].*** *"Groups did not differ in the THC content of the cannabis they smoked. Unlike the marked impairment in prose recall of individuals who smoked cannabis low in cannabidiol, participants smoking cannabis high in cannabidiol showed no memory impairment."*

I read a, dubiously, scientific article that suggests that during the "high" insuced by cannabis consumption, THC causes a disruption in short term memory and the ability to commit something to long term memory. However, I think many cannabis users would disagree and I disagree as well.

For this to be true, the subject would have to be really really high, almost in a state of comatose, which would mean ingesting a dosage of THC well above the tolerance level, which is currently set at about 50mg per day.

I, also believe that for this research to be validated, other factors would have to be taken into consideration like: the subject's age, their mindfulness at the time of consumption and their current mental capacity for committing to memory and memory recall. If someone already has poor memory, they will clearly still have poor memory while ingesting cannabis. Having said that, according to an article published by the Telegraph, Ohio State University, *"found that specific elements of marijuana can be good for the ageing brain by reducing inflammation there and possibly even stimulating the formation of new brain cells. The research suggests that the development of a legal drug that contains certain properties similar to those in marijuana might help prevent or delay the onset of Alzheimer's disease."*

Myth No. 2 - Using Cannabis leads to cancer

Fact -   Cannabinoids found in Cannabis have
                been proven to shrink tumours.

According to the Medical News Today, research
carried out at Complutense University in Spain,
*"THC induced the death of brain cancer cells in a
process known as "autophagy. When human tumors
in mice were targeted with doses of THC, the
researchers found that two cell receptors were
particularly associated with an anti-tumor
response. The researchers found that administering
THC to mice with human tumors initiated
autophagy and caused the growth of the tumors to
decrease. Two human patients with highly
aggressive brain tumors who received intracranial
administration of THC also showed similar signs of
autophagy, upon analysis."*

Myth No. 3 - Cannabis users are drug addicts.

Fact -   Physiologically, cannabis contains no
                addictive chemical substances what so
                ever.

What is addictive is the tobacco some users mix
with the cannabis when they smoke it. Tobacco is a
seriously addictive substance and hazardous to your
health - not cannabis.

I doubt this would ever happen but, if a cannabis user claimed to be addicted, it's more likely they are "psychologically" hooked on the high, or the feeling of tranquility, that they get from the THC. This would imply they already have some form of "addictive" personality. So, many psychological factors would have to be taken into account before any study could prove cannabis addiction.

As a final note, I know several people who only ever smoke one joint a day, before bed. It helps them to relax, meditate better and improve their quality of sleep. During the day, they function perfectly normally. They don't crave a joint nor are they addicted. In fact, they can go long periods without using cannabis at all and have no side effects nor cravings.

Myth No. 4 - The use of Cannabis leads to criminal behaviour

Fact -   Because of the way cannabis affects the mind and body, people on a high from the THC content are, quite frankly, too zoned out or "happy" to behave criminally.

It's probably fairer to say that the use of cannabis is high among criminals and not that cannabis causes criminal behaviour. It's a well documented fact that there are more criminal activities and acts of aggression through alcohol consumption than the use of cannabis.

Furthermore, in Colorado, it's reported that crime went down 14,6% since the legalisation of cannabis. Prior to that, the main criminal activities, related to cannabis, were growing, driving while under the influence, possession and selling.

Myth No. 5 - Cannabis users spend their whole time spaced out.

Fact -   That's the most absurd statement I've ever heard.

That's like saying all drinkers spend their whole day drunk. While people may enjoy social drinking, it only really takes over your life when you become an alcoholic. Similarly, while, no doubt, there are people in the world who make frequent   recreational use   of cannabis, or perhaps abuse its consumption, medical use of cannabis will not space you out all day. For that to happen, you'd have to take very high quantities at very frequent   intervals.

The use of cannabis, like medication, alcohol, food etc. should be used in moderation; according to each individual's need and tolerance. If you've never taken cannabis before, you should not try and down a whole teaspoon of cannabis oil in your first sitting. You should start with less than a quarter of a teaspoon and gradually allow your tolerance levels to build over time.

6 CANNABIS TEA

As I mentioned earlier, you don't have to smoke cannabis. There are many other ways to consume the plant without inhaling it. One such way is through drinking it as a tea and when you do, the effects are much milder than with any other form of consumption.

Since new scientific evidence is coming to light every day regarding the beneficial properties of this plant, nobody truly knows its full capabilities. However, some of the benefits of drinking a cannabis infused tea are: relieving anxiety, inducing a state of relaxation, alleviating chronic pain and reducing nausea.

According to the Society for the confluence of festivals in India, cannabis, or bhang as it's known, *"If taken in proper quantity bhang cures fever, dysentery and sunstroke. It helps to clear phlegm, quicken digestion, sharpen appetite, cure speak imperfection and lispering. Besides, it freshens the intellect and gives alertness to the body and gaiety to the mind."*

In fact, the earliest known cannabis infusions probably originated in India where it is still considered a sacred drink linked to the God Shiva. Dating back as far as 1000 AD or earlier, bhang was given to guests to test their religiosity and their loyalty to their hosts. It is, also, still very much used during sacred festivals.

As the story goes, Shiva, a Hindu Deity, was very angry and out walking one day when he stopped to take shelter, from the sun, under a cannabis plant. Not knowing what it was, he ate the leaves and felt his anxiety and anger lift. He claimed to meditate better and felt more transcendental clarity. After his experience, he shared his knowledge with everyone around him. To this day, he is still referred to as the God of Bhang.

In India, Bhang is prepared by making a pesto of the cannabis leaves and buds and then adding to that hot milk, spices and ghee, which is similar to butter in the west. You might even try adding a teaspoon of honey into the mix.

Another popular way to make a cannabis infusion is by grinding up the cannabis leaves and buds, in a coffee grinder for example, and then placing the contents into an empty tea bag. Bring some water to boil in a saucepan and then reduce the heat, add a little butter, milk, coconut milk or coconut oil and pop the tea bag in the saucepan. Let it simmer on a lower temperature for about 20 minutes. Remove it from the heat and allow it to sit for about another 45 minutes before consuming.

Another idea might be to mix the cannabis leaves and/or bud with another tea, like lemongrass for example. Place the lemongrass and the cannabis into a tea pot, add hot water and let it sit for a while before consuming it. Again, you can sweeten to your liking.

One very important thing you should know is that THC is a fat soluble substance. What does this mean? It means that if you do not put oil of some kind, or butter or ghee, into your tea, the effects will be minimal to non existent, because water alone does not separate the THC from the leaves.

7 CANNABIS OINTMENT

Cannabis ointment, or salve or topic as some may refer to it, is very easy to make. You can do it by mixing together 2 cups of marijuana with 2 cups of coconut oil and roughly 56 grams of pure beeswax. To give it a more pleasant aroma, you might like to add into the mix an essential oil of your choice. Lavender is often a good choice because it has its own healing and soothing properties.

The way to make the oil is as follows:

Start off by putting the cannabis into the oven on a tray at about 200 degrees for about 20 minutes. This is to decarboxylate the plant. In layman's terms, decarboxylation means toasting the plant to activate its THC content and get the most out of its healing properties. The cannabis should be spread nice and evenly on the tray and you should turn it over every now and then to ensure all parts brown up equally. Once its ready, remove it from the oven and grind it a little in a coffee grinder.

While the cannabis is in the oven, put the coconut oil in a pan, on the stove, on a very low heat.

Add the ground cannabis to the oil and let it simmer for about 20 minutes. When you remove the cannabis infused oil from the stove, you will want to filter it by using something like a cheese cloth; to remove all parts of the plant. Make sure you wring the cloth well to get all the oil out.

Then, in a separate saucepan melt the beeswax. Once melted, you can add your cannabis infused coconut oil to it and whatever essential oil you have chosen. Let it set and cool a little. Then pour into a jar. Once it's completely cooled down, it will start to solidify and you can store it in the fridge.

If you want to potentiate your cannabis oil and give it extra beneficial healing properties, while it's still warm, you can add to it 1 tablespoon of magnesium chloride.

Magnesium chloride is essential for the human body but nowadays, the majority of people suffer with magnesium deficiency due to poor diets high in refined sugars and processed foods. Magnesium deficiency leads to all kinds of problems such as coronary disease, mental depression, irritability and insomnia; among others.

Sadly, due to over farming, the use of pesticides, soil condition and genetic modification of food, fruit and vegetables, we buy nowadays, only contain traces of magnesium or they are completely void of it.

Studies have shown how magnesium benefits the prevention of cancer and how it can be used as a cure for the disease. According to the study: *MAGNESIUM IN ONCOGENESIS AND IN ANTI-CANCER TREATMENT: INTERACTION WITH MINERALS AND VITAMINS*, regions where there is a greater magnesium deficiency have a higher number of cases of cancer.

"A Russian report showed that stomach cancer is four times more common (40/100,000) in the Ukraine where the Mg content of soil and drinking water is low, than it is in Armenia (10/100,000) where the Mg content is more than twice as high.(14,66-68) A more recent morphologic and statistical analysis of neoplastic deaths in two Polish communities(69) disclosed a nearly three-fold higher death rate in the one in a low soil Mg area (27%) than in the one with high soil Mg (10%). The malignancies accounting for the differences were mainly adeno- and squamous cell carcinomas in the gastrointestinal tract (61.3%) and respiratory system (22.3%)."

Although magnesium can be safely ingested, it can, also, be used externally by being applied to the skin in an oil form. It gets absorbed through the pores of the skin.

So, what are the uses of cannabis ointment?

You can use it for massage to help relieve aches and pains and tensions in the body. You can use it on scrapes, cuts, boils and insect bites. In some cases it's effective against itchiness of the skin. It, also, proved to be effective in the treatment of acne; according to a study published by the Journal of Clinical Investigation.

At present, there are no real scientific research conclusions, that I could find, relating to the efficacy of cannabis ointment and the treatment of more chronic skin conditions such as psoriasis and eczema. The good news is, with the new legal laws regarding cannabis, new investigations in this area are being conducted so it won't be long before we have news from the medical field. More good news is, there are plenty of testimonials online, by psoriasis sufferers, who claim that cannabis has helped them tremendously in some way or another. There are also supportive articles by naturopathic doctors.

Finally, the 2014 investigation: *Involvement of the endocannabinoid system in osteoarthritis pain* suggests cannabinoids show *"promising results that*

*have been recently obtained in support of the
therapeutic value of cannabinoids for osteoarthritis
management."*

8 CANNABIS OIL

The process to make cannabis oil, for ingestion, is very similar to the process you would use to produce the ointment without the beeswax. In fact, you can make both at the same time from one single batch of cannabis and coconut oil. Again, you can use a ratio of roughly 2 cups of marijuana to 2 cups of pure, extra virgin, organic coconut oil.

The preparation procedure is basically the same. You start off by placing the cannabis into the oven on a tray at about 200 degrees for about 20 minutes to decarboxylate the plant. I explained this in the previous section. The cannabis should be spread nice and evenly on the tray and you should turn it over every now and then to ensure all parts brown up equally. Once its ready, remove it from the oven and grind it a little in a coffee grinder.

The infusing process is a little different. In fact, while the cannabis is in the oven, the coconut oil should be placed in a slow cook pot, on low temperature, and allowed to melt slowly.

At this point, when you have the ground cannabis, you want to package it up in some cheesecloth and make sure it can't get out into the oil.

Add the package of ground cannabis to the oil, in the slow cook pot, and let it sit there on the low temperature for about 4 to 5 hours. Make sure the package soaks up all the coconut oil. Every hour or so, you need to turn the package over to ensure all the properties of the cannabis infuse into the oil.

After the 4 or 5 hours what you should have is a green to light brown oil. When you remove the package make sure you wring it well to get all the oil out. Ideally, you should use clean latex (or other material) gloves for this process.

At this point, as mentioned in a earlier section, you can add magnesium to the oil to potentiate its effects.

You now have two choices. You can either fill empty gel capsules with the oil; using a droplet pipette or you can place the oil in a jar and use it, as and when needed, by adding it to your cooking.

A very important word of caution. Whichever way you choose to use it, go easy on the dosage you ingest. If you're using capsules, take one a day and preferably at a time when you're not going to be doing anything. If you're adding it to cooking, make sure it's also at a time when you won't be doing much. You will get a high. So, depending on your tolerance level, your capacity to drive, for example, will be impaired.

If you're using a teaspoon to dose a serving, start with 1/4 of a teaspoon and increase very modestly until you find the quantity that suits your tolerance level. Remember, the aim is to provide the body with supportive healing and not turn yourselves into a "non compos mentis" zombie.

You should also be aware that, depending on your metabolic rate, it can take up to 40 minutes to feel the high from the ingested cannabis. So, just because you have no immediate effects after ingestion, does not mean that you will not have them. So, don't go taking more and   more.

9 JUICING RAW CANNABIS LEAVES

Juicing raw cannabis leaves has many beneficial properties for good health. It's antioxidant and anti-inflammatory and the great news is, for those people who don't want the "high" that comes from heating cannabis, there is NO high.

It's absolutely no different to juicing kale or wheatgrass, for example. However, you can still benefit from the cannabinoid content of the plant.

Cannabis leaves are pretty much like any green leafy vegetable. They are full of rich nutrients such as: iron, calcium and fiber. Once you juice the leaves, the fiber is broken down.

The juicing process is very easy. You collect about 10 to 15 large sized cannabis leaves, wash them thoroughly and put them through a good juicer.

Once you have extracted the juice, it's ready for drinking. As with all fresh juices, for optimum benefits, you should drink it within 20 minutes of juicing.

Some people find cannabis juice has a bitter taste. So, you may want to add in a little fruit or vegetable juice of your choosing. While you have your juicer at hand, it's a great idea to make your own fresh juice to add into the mix. A suggestion might be fresh apple juice.

However, if you're buying a pre-packaged juice to add in to the mix, make sure it's 100% pure fruit and not made from 100% fruit concentrate, which has no beneficial properties what so ever for good health. Once a fruit has been turned into a concentrate, it loses its rich nutrients such as: vitamins, minerals, folic acid, carotenes, fiber and so forth.

If you would like to know more about fruit concentrate and its process, you can find plenty of resources online.

Appendix

Cannabis kills tumor cells

- http://www.ncbi.nlm.nih.gov/pmc/articles/PMC1576089

- http://www.ncbi.nlm.nih.gov/pubmed/20090845

- http://www.ncbi.nlm.nih.gov/pubmed/616322

- http://www.ncbi.nlm.nih.gov/pubmed/14640910

Uterine, testicular, and pancreatic cancers

- http://www.cancer.gov/cancertopics/pdq/cam/cannabis/healthprofessional/page4

- http://www.ncbi.nlm.nih.gov/pubmed/20925 645

Brain cancer

- http://www.ncbi.nlm.nih.gov/pubmed/11479 216

Mouth and throat cancer

- http://www.ncbi.nlm.nih.gov/pubmed/20516 734

Breast cancer

- http://www.ncbi.nlm.nih.gov/pubmed/18454 173

- http://www.ncbi.nlm.nih.gov/pubmed/16728 591

- http://www.ncbi.nlm.nih.gov/pubmed/96531 94

Lung cancer

- http://www.ncbi.nlm.nih.gov/pubmed/25069 049

- http://www.ncbi.nlm.nih.gov/pubmed/22198 381?dopt=Abstract

- http://www.ncbi.nlm.nih.gov/pubmed/21097 714?dopt=Abstract

Prostate cancer

- http://www.ncbi.nlm.nih.gov/pubmed/12746 841?dopt=Abstract

- http://www.ncbi.nlm.nih.gov/pmc/articles/P MC3339795/?tool=pubmed

- http://www.ncbi.nlm.nih.gov/pubmed/22594 963

- http://www.ncbi.nlm.nih.gov/pubmed/15753 356

Blood cancer

- http://www.ncbi.nlm.nih.gov/pubmed/12091 357

- http://www.ncbi.nlm.nih.gov/pubmed/16908 594

Skin cancer

- http://www.ncbi.nlm.nih.gov/pubmed/12511587

- http://www.ncbi.nlm.nih.gov/pubmed/19608284

Liver cancer

- http://www.ncbi.nlm.nih.gov/pubmed/21475304

Cannabis cancer cures (general)

- http://www.ncbi.nlm.nih.gov/pubmed/12514108

- http://www.ncbi.nlm.nih.gov/pubmed/15313899

- http://www.ncbi.nlm.nih.gov/pubmed/20053780

- http://www.ncbi.nlm.nih.gov/pubmed/18199524

Cancers of the head and neck

- http://ww.ncbi.nlm.nih.gov/pmc/articles/PMC2277494

Cholangiocarcinoma cancer

- http://ww.ncbi.nlm.nih.gov/pubmed/19916793

- http://www.ncbi.nlm.nih.gov/pubmed/21115947

Leukemia

- http://www.ncbi.nlm.nih.gov/pubmed/15454482

- http://www.ncbi.nlm.nih.gov/pubmed/16139274

- http://www.ncbi.nlm.nih.gov/pubmed/14692532

Cannabis partially/fully induced cancer cell death

- http://www.ncbi.nlm.nih.gov/pubmed/12130702

- http://www.ncbi.nlm.nih.gov/pubmed/19457575

- http://www.ncbi.nlm.nih.gov/pubmed/18615 640

- http://www.ncbi.nlm.nih.gov/pubmed/17931 597

- http://www.ncbi.nlm.nih.gov/pubmed/18438 336

- http://www.ncbi.nlm.nih.gov/pubmed/19916 793

Translocation-positive rhabdomyosarcoma

- http://www.ncbi.nlm.nih.gov/pubmed/19509 271

Lymphoma

- http://www.ncbi.nlm.nih.gov/pubmed/18546 271

- http://www.ncbi.nlm.nih.gov/pubmed/16936 228

- http://www.ncbi.nlm.nih.gov/pubmed/16337 199

-

- http://www.ncbi.nlm.nih.gov/pubmed/19609004

Cannabis kills cancer cells

- http://www.ncbi.nlm.nih.gov/pubmed/16818634

- http://www.ncbi.nlm.nih.gov/pubmed/12648025

- http://www.ncbi.nlm.nih.gov/pubmed/17952650

- http://www.ncbi.nlm.nih.gov/pubmed/16835997

Melanoma

- http://www.ncbi.nlm.nih.gov/pubmed/17065222

Thyroid carcinoma

- http://www.ncbi.nlm.nih.gov/pubmed/18197164

Colon cancer

- http://www.ncbi.nlm.nih.gov/pubmed/18938775

- http://www.ncbi.nlm.nih.gov/pubmed/19047095

Intestinal inflammation and cancer

- http://www.ncbi.nlm.nih.gov/pubmed/19442536

Cannabinoids in health and disease

- http://www.ncbi.nlm.nih.gov/pubmed/18286801

Cannabis inhibits cancer cell invasion

- http://www.ncbi.nlm.nih.gov/pubmed/19914218

Bibliography and References:

WHO | Diabetes
http://www.who.int/mediacentre/factsheets/fs312/en
/

WHO | Pharmaceutical Industry
www.who.int/trade/glossary/story073/en/

Open Secrets
http://www.opensecrets.org/industries/indus.php?in
d=h04

Forbes
http://www.forbes.com/forbes/welcome/

Persecuted (and murdered) doctors, health
professionals
http://www.whale.to/a/persecuted_doc_h.html

Complete Health and Happiness
http://complete-health-and-
happiness.com/cannabinoid-oil-saves-babys-life-by-
dissolving-brain-tumor-after-family-rejects-
chemotherapy/

Visiongain
https://www.visiongain.com/Press_Release/405/Dia
betes-drugs-market-will-reach-55-3bn-in-2017-

with-further-growth-to-2023-predicts-visiongain-in-new-report

Marihuana: The First Twelve Thousand Years"
Ernest L Abel, 1980
http://files.meetup.com/18500005/Abel.%20marihu
ana%20the%20first%20twelve%20thousand%20ye
ars.pdf

Independent Drug Monitoring Unit
http://www.idmu.co.uk/historical.htm

Thrillist
https://www.thrillist.com/vice/30-places-where-weed-is-legal-cities-and-countries-with-decriminalized-marijuana

Neuroscience. 2nd edition.
Purves D, Augustine GJ, Fitzpatrick D, et al.,
editors.
Sunderland (MA): Sinauer Associates; 2001.

Science Explains How Cannabis Kills Cancer Cells
| CBD-Healthcare News
https://www.youtube.com/watch?v=5RtRil2ND-E

Society for the confluence of Festivals in India
http://www.holifestival.org/tradition-of-bhang.html

Medicinal Marijuana Association
http://www.medicinalmarijuanaassociation.com/me
dical-marijuana-blog/3-lessons-learned-about-cannabis-tea

The journal of Clinical Investigation
https://www.jci.org/articles/view/64628

Involvement of the endocannabinoid system in
osteoarthritis pain.
European Journal of Neuroscience 2014 Feb.
La Porta C. Bura SA. Negrete R. Maldonado R.
http://www.ncbi.nlm.nih.gov/pubmed/24494687

Cannabidiol for neurodegenerative disorders:
important new clinical applications for this
phytocannabinoid?
Javier Fernández-Ruiz,[1,2,3] Onintza Sagredo,[1,2,3] M
Ruth Pazos,[4] Concepción García,[1,2,3] Roger
Pertwee,[5] Raphael Mechoulam,[6] and José Martínez-
Orgado[4,7]
Br J Clin Pharmacol. 2013 Feb; 75(2): 323–333.
Published online 2012 May 25. doi:
10.1111/j.1365-2125.2012.04341.x
http://www.ncbi.nlm.nih.gov/pubmed/22625422

Impact of cannabidiol on the acute memory and
psychotomimetic effects of smoked cannabis:
naturalistic study: naturalistic study [corrected].
Morgan CJ[1], Schafer G, Freeman TP, Curran HV.
Br J Psychiatry. 2010 Oct;197(4):285-90. doi:
10.1192/bjp.bp.110.077503.
http://www.ncbi.nlm.nih.gov/pubmed/20884951

Marijuana may improve memory and help fight
Alzheimer's
The Telegraph - Richard Alleyne, Science
Correspondent

19 Nov 2008
http://www.telegraph.co.uk/news/science/science-news/3485163/Marijuana-may-improve-memory-and-help-fight-Alzheimers.html

Cannabis reduces tumor growth in study
Written by David McNamee
Last reviewed: Mon 13 July 2015
http://www.medicalnewstoday.com/articles/279571.php

Magnesium in oncogenesis and in anti-cancer treatment: Interaction with minerals and vitamins.
Mildred S. Seelig, M.D., M.P.H.
In Adjuvant Nutrition in Cancer Treatment, Eds. P. Quillan and R. M. Williams. Publ Cancer Treatment Research Foundation, 1993. Chapt. 15:238-318.
http://www.mgwater.com/cancer.shtml

Cannabinoids inhibit neurodegeneration in models of multiple sclerosis
Gareth Pryce, Zubair Ahmed, Deborah J. R. Hankey, Samuel J. Jackson, J. Ludovic Croxford, Jennifer M. Pocock, Catherine Ledent, Axel Petzold, Alan J. Thompson, Gavin Giovannoni, M. Louise Cuzner, David Baker
DOI: http://dx.doi.org/10.1093/brain/awg224

Diverse functions of ceramide in cancer cell death and proliferation.

Saddoughi SA[1], Ogretmen B
http://www.ncbi.nlm.nih.gov/pubmed/23290776

How Cannabis Oil Works to Kill Cancer Cells
Dennis Hill
http://www.cureyourowncancer.org/how-cannabis-oil-works.html#sthash.IA04zKZO.dpuf

Neuroprotective effects of phytocannabinoid-based medicines in experimental models of Huntington's disease.
Sagredo O[1], Pazos MR, Satta V, Ramos JA, Pertwee RG, Fernández-Ruiz J.
http://www.ncbi.nlm.nih.gov/pubmed/21674569

Cannabis (medical marijuana) treatment for motor and non-motor symptoms of Parkinson disease: an open-label observational study.
(http://www.ncbi.nlm.nih.gov/pubmed/24614667)

CBD improves well-being and quality of life in Parkinson's disease patients.
Effects of cannabidiol in the treatment of patients with Parkinson's disease: an exploratory double-blind trial.
(http://www.ncbi.nlm.nih.gov/pubmed/25237116

Epilepsy Foundation Colorado
The Use of Cannabis to Treat Children with Epilepsy
Updated February 2016
http://www.epilepsycolorado.org/news-research/medical-marijuana/efco-report-to-the-

community/

Safety and Efficacy of Medical Cannabis Oil for Behavioral and Psychological Symptoms of Dementia: An-Open Label, Add-On, Pilot Study. Shelef A[1], Barak Y[1], Berger U[2], Paleacu D[1], Tadger S[1], Plopsky I[1], Baruch Y[1].
http://www.ncbi.nlm.nih.gov/pubmed/26757043

American Academy of Ophthalmology
Written by: David Turbert, contributing writer: Dayle Kern
Reviewed by: Dr. J. Kevin McKinney, MD, MPH
Jun. 27, 2014
http://www.aao.org/eye-health/tips-prevention/medical-marijuana-glaucoma-treament

MY PRAYER FOR YOU ALL

May you always have happiness and the causes of
happiness
May you always have good health and the causes for good
health
May you never suffer nor those you love.
May all causes of suffering be removed from your life.
Live, Love and be happy!
Life really is too short!